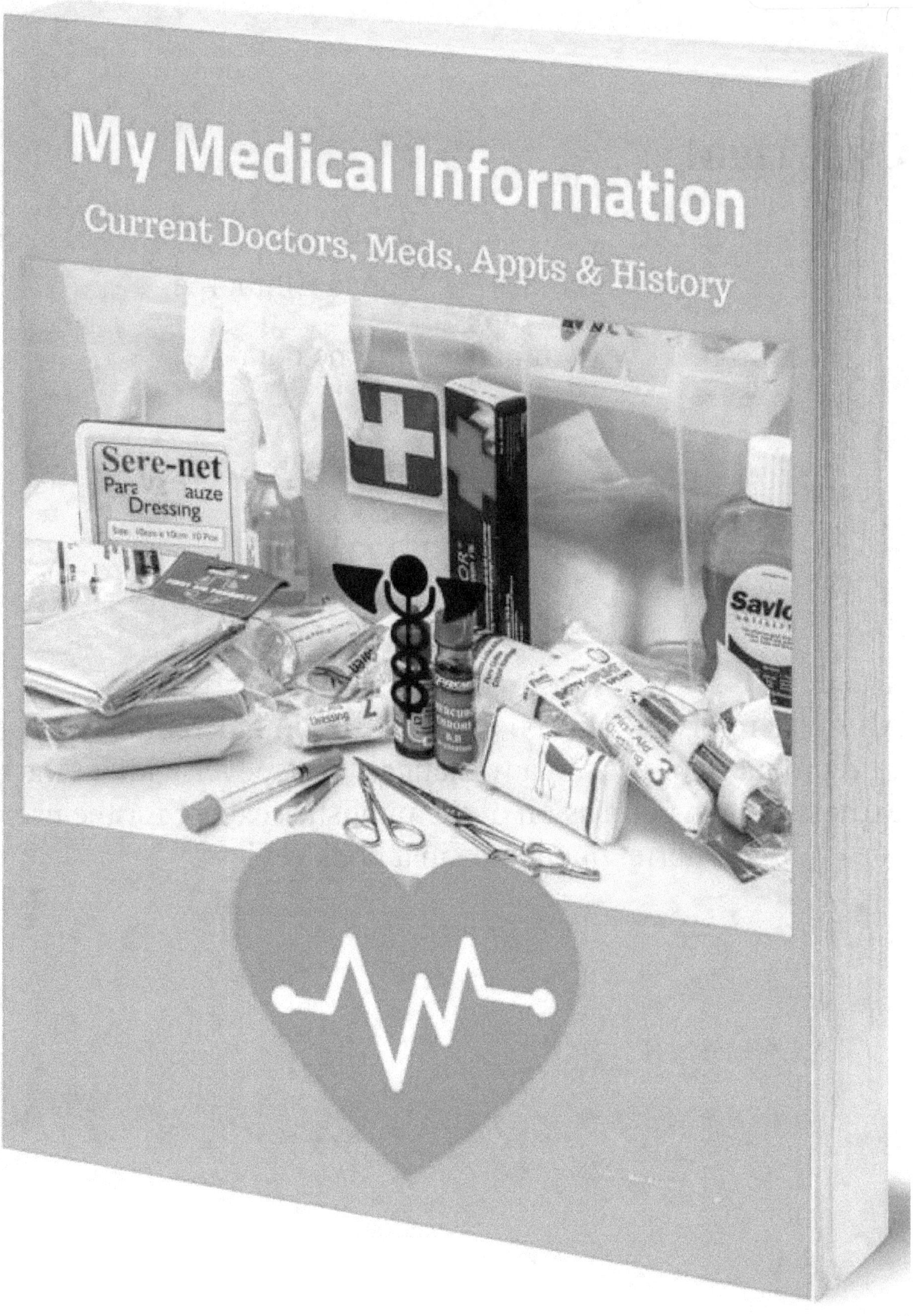

My Medical Information
Current Doctors, Meds, Appts & History

Copyright

MEDICAL DISCLAIMER

Disclaimer and Terms of Use: No information contained in this book should be considered as physical, health related, financial, tax, or legal advice. Your reliance upon information and content obtained by you at or through this publication is solely at your own risk. The author assumes no liability or responsibly for damage or injury to you, other persons, or property arising from any use of any product, information, idea, or instruction contained in the content provided to you through this book.

Always remember if there is an emergency call 9-1-1 and not wait on a return call from your doctor.

CONTENTS

Patient Information

Name:
Address:
Home Phone:
Cell:
Email:

Emergency Contacts:

Name/Phone:
Name/Phone:
Name/Phone:

Personal Patient Information:

Birth Date:
Height:
Weight:
Blood Type
Ethnicity/Race:

Family Medical History

Diseases / Illnesses Known
Mother:
Father:
Brothers:
Sisters:
Grandmothers:
Grandfathers:
Relatives:

Family Medical History

Diseases / Illnesses Known

Medication Log

ALLERGIES
Prescription:
Dosage:
Frequency:
Prescription Date:
Doctor:
Prescription:
Dosage:
Frequency:
Prescription Date:
Doctor:

Medication Log

ALLERGIES
Prescription:
Dosage:
Frequency:
Prescription Date:
Doctor:
Prescription:
Dosage:
Frequency:
Prescription Date:
Doctor:

Medication Log

ALLERGIES
Prescription:
Dosage:
Frequency:
Prescription Date:
Doctor:
Prescription:
Dosage:
Frequency:
Prescription Date:
Doctor:

Medication Log

ALLERGIES
Prescription:
Dosage:
Frequency:
Prescription Date:
Doctor:
Prescription:
Dosage:
Frequency:
Prescription Date:
Doctor:

Medication Log

ALLERGIES
Prescription:
Dosage:
Frequency:
Prescription Date:
Doctor:
Prescription:
Dosage:
Frequency:
Prescription Date:
Doctor:

Vaccination Record

Vaccine	Date:

Vaccination Record

Vaccine	Date:

NOTES

NOTES

Insurance

Provider Name:
Address:
Phone:
Email:
Website:
Policy Number:
ID/Member Number:

Notes:

Notes:

Doctor:

Name:	
Phone No.:	
Address:	
Appointment Date:	
Appointment Time:	
Reason For Visit:	
Diagnosis:	
Treatment:	
Tests Ordered:	
Medication:	
Follow-up Date:	
Doctor Referral:	
NOTES:	

Notes:

Notes:

Specialist:

Name:	
Phone No.:	
Address:	
Appointment Date:	
Appointment Time:	
Reason For Visit:	
Diagnosis:	
Treatment:	
Tests Ordered:	
Medication:	
Follow-up Appointment Date:	
Follow-up Appointment Time:	
Doctor Referral:	

Notes:

Notes:

Surgeon:

Name:	
Phone No.:	
Address:	
Appointment Date:	
Appointment Time:	
Reason For Visit:	
Diagnosis:	
Treatment:	
Tests Ordered:	
Medication:	
Follow-up Appointment Date and Time:	
Doctor Referral:	

Notes:

Notes:

Lab Work:

Name:	
Phone No.:	
Address:	
Appointment Date and Time:	
Lab Work Ordered:	
Ordered By:	
Results:	

Lab Work:

Name:	
Phone No.:	
Address:	
Appointment Date and Time:	
Lab Work Ordered:	
Ordered By:	
Results:	

Lab Work:

Name:	
Phone No.:	
Address:	
Appointment Date and Time:	
Lab Work Ordered:	
Ordered By:	
Results:	

Lab Work:

Name:	
Phone No.:	
Address:	
Appointment Date and Time:	
Lab Work Ordered:	
Ordered By:	
Results:	

Lab Work:

Name:
Phone No.:
Address:
Appointment Date and Time:
Lab Work Ordered:
Ordered By:
Results:

Lab Work:

Name:	
Phone No.:	
Address:	
Appointment Date and Time:	
Lab Work Ordered:	
Ordered By:	
Results:	

X-rays:

Name:	
Phone No.:	
Address:	
Appointment Date and Time:	
Xrays Ordered:	
Ordered By:	
Results:	

X-rays:

Name:
Phone No.:
Address:
Appointment Date and Time:
Xrays Ordered:
Ordered By:
Results:

X-rays:

Name:	
Phone No.:	
Address:	
Appointment Date and Time:	
Xrays Ordered:	
Ordered By:	
Results:	

X-rays:

Name:	
Phone No.:	
Address:	
Appointment Date and Time:	
Xrays Ordered:	
Ordered By:	
Results:	

Notes:

Notes:

Respiratory Therapy:

Name:
Phone No.:
Address:
Appointment Date and Time:
Therapist:
Treatment:
Results:

Respiratory Therapy:

Name:	
Phone No.:	
Address:	
Appointment Date and Time:	
Therapist:	
Treatment:	
Results:	

Respiratory Therapy:

Name:	
Phone No.:	
Address:	
Appointment Date and Time:	
Therapist:	
Treatment:	
Results:	

Respiratory Therapy:

Name:
Phone No.:
Address:
Appointment Date and Time:
Therapist:
Treatment:
Results:

Notes:

Notes:

Notes:

Notes:

Notes:

Notes:

Notes:

Notes:

Notes:

Notes:

Notes:

Notes:

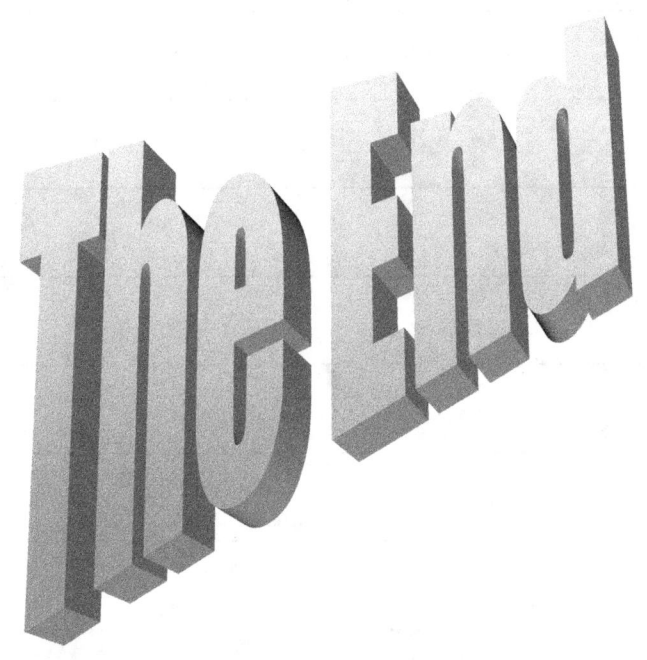

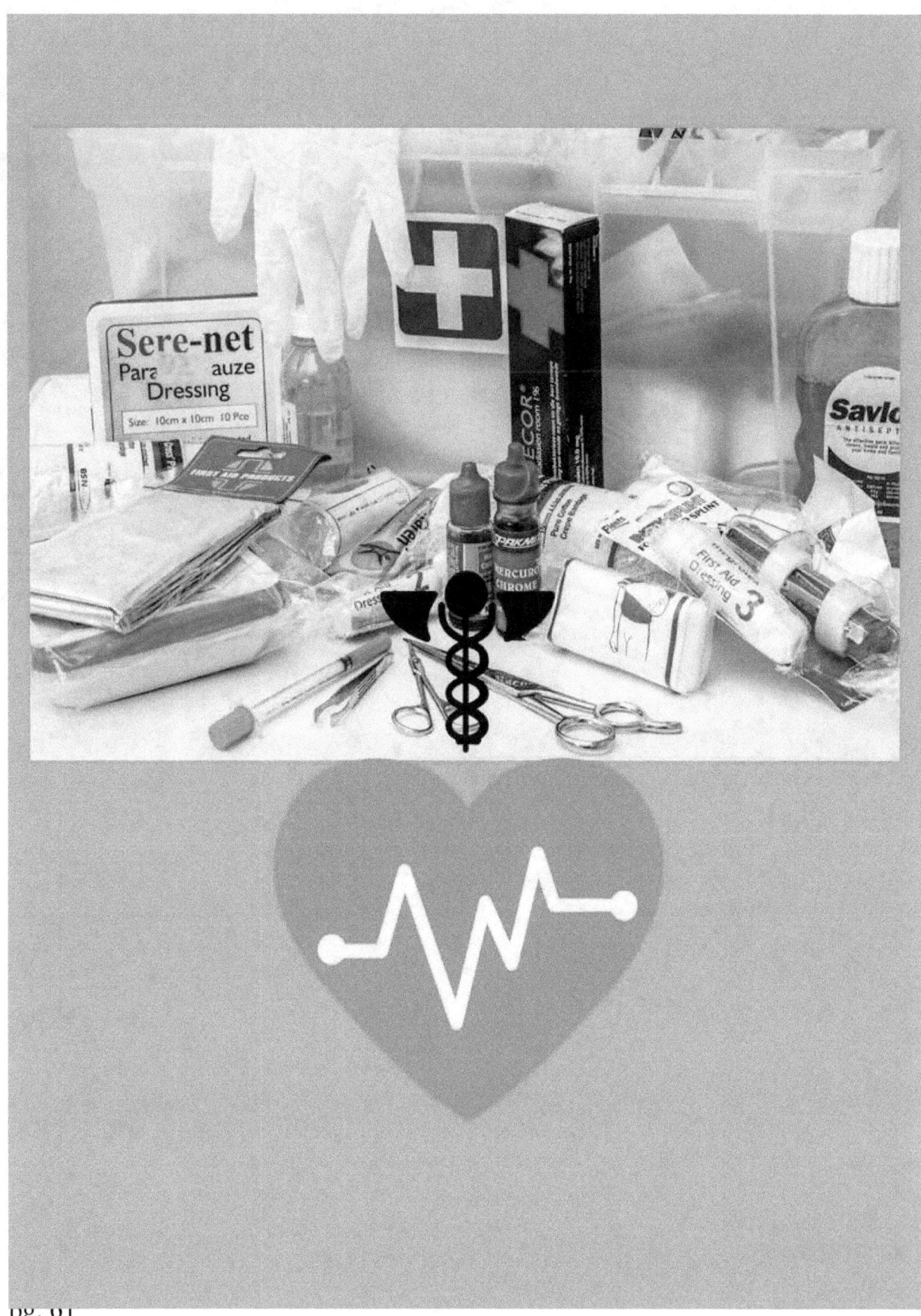

www.ingramcontent.com/pod-product-compliance
Lightning Source LLC
Chambersburg PA
CBHW081618220526
45468CB00010B/2929